PET CARE
Handbooks

THE
HEALTHY
AQUARIUM

**Dr Roger Sweeting
and Dr Anne Powell**

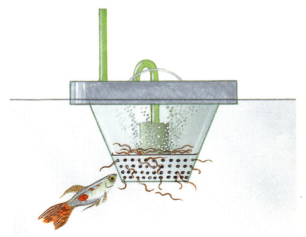

HAMLYN

Published by
The Hamlyn Publishing Group Limited
A division of The Octopus Publishing Group plc
Michelin House, 81 Fulham Road,
London SW3 6RB, England
and distributed for them by
Octopus Distribution Services Limited
Rushden, Northamptonshire NN10 9RZ, England

First published 1988

ISBN 0 600 55751 0

Some of the material in this book
is reproduced from other books published
by the Hamlyn Publishing Group Limited.

Printed by Mandarin Offset, Hong Kong

Contents

Introduction

The fish in your aquarium or pond depend on you for a healthy life. To keep them free of diseases you must house them properly and feed them the right amount of good food. You must also keep their water clean and not crowd too many fish in one small tank or pond. You must learn about your fish so that you recognize when they are unwell and if they do become ill or diseased you must know how to treat them.

It is hoped that you will never have any sick fish. This book explains how to make sure that your fish stay healthy, but if, despite all your efforts to give your fish the best possible environment, they still become ill, some of the diseases that can affect them and how you should treat them have been described. Do not forget, treating a sick fish is a last resort. The best way to ensure that your fish live to a ripe old age is to look after them well, so that they do not become ill.

There are some diseases that are not easily treatable. For these you will need to consult a veterinary surgeon

Below: *points to look for in a healthy fish*
Right: *healthy congo salmon*

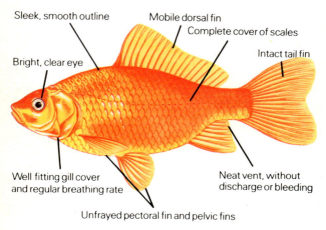

Sleek, smooth outline

Mobile dorsal fin

Complete cover of scales

Intact tail fin

Bright, clear eye

Well fitting gill cover and regular breathing rate

Neat vent, without discharge or bleeding

Unfrayed pectoral fin and pelvic fins

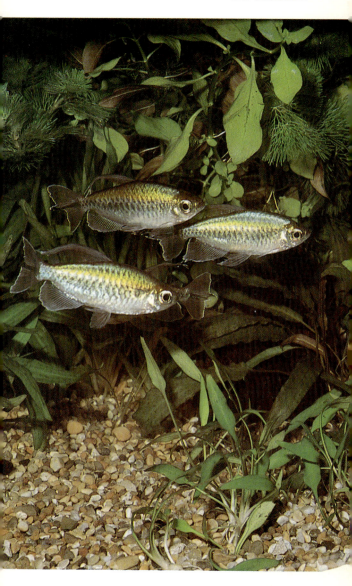

or fish pathologist. Our knowledge of fish diseases is much less than that of diseases of mammals or of people, so that when fish do become ill, there is a much greater chance that successful treatment will not be available.

How long do fish live?

What is old age for fish and how long should we expect them to live? Small tropical fish and small goldfish may live for only 18 months. Larger koi or goldfish can live for much longer, often as long as 10 or 15 years, and large carp, oscars and groupers for 40 years. Usually the bigger the fish the longer you can expect it to live. Although some fish can live for many years most die long before from infections brought on by the stress of a poor environment.

Very few fish die of old age. Normally as they get older and become weaker they are overcome by one of the many disease-causing organisms that abound in every pond. These harmful organisms include bacteria, fungi and a range of animal parasites such as flukes and tapeworms.

Carp tapeworm: found in the intestine of grass carp and koi

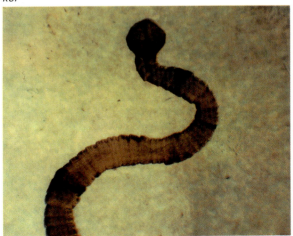

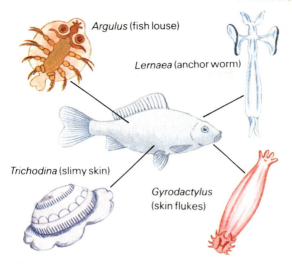

Argulus (fish louse)

Lernaea (anchor worm)

Trichodina (slimy skin)

Gyrodactylus (skin flukes)

Four of the commonest ectoparasites of freshwater fish. Each of these parasites can kill the fish when present in large numbers

In temperate climates it is possible to tell the age of a fish by examining its scales with a lens or a microscope. The scales resemble cross sections of tree rings in that there are concentric circles from the centre to the edge. These rings develop as the fish grows so that the same number of scales still adequately covers the whole body. In fast growth the rings are far apart, in slow growth they are close together. During the winter when fish stop growing altogether there is a pronounced break in the arrangement of these rings, which means the fish's age in years can be assessed. Fish kept under constant conditions of temperature and food will not show pronounced annual rings.

Fish with a health problem may stop growing so under these circumstances a growth check can be seen. When fish lose scales through damage, secondary scales are quickly created to replace those lost. Unlike the original or primary scales these are thrown together so that no neat rings of growth can be seen. When they reach the same size as the original scales they begin to grow in a neat, ordered fashion. An examination of the scales of fish can therefore provide quite a detailed insight into the history of that fish.

Unlike most other vertebrates fish grow throughout life and do not have a final adult size. Growth slows down as they get older and very old fish may even start to lose weight.

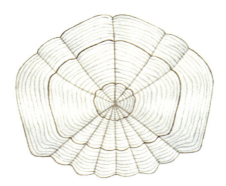

Fish scale to show fine rings (circuli) and annual rings (annuli). Annual rings indicate the cessation of growth in the winter followed by an increase in growth in the spring. Fish in constant conditions may not form annual rings

Sometimes very old fish can be recognized by their appearance alone; they are thin, their scales show considerable irregularities and they hang listlessly in the water unless disturbed. Such fish should be avoided as they will not do well or breed.

Preventing disease

Healthy stock

In a new tank there are two ways in which parasites and diseases can be introduced to your fish. Firstly, the fish you buy may already be diseased. You can avoid this by buying fish from a good dealer.

Even good dealers cannot give health guarantees, however, and it is unreasonable to expect them to, even with really expensive fish. There are several points that can be used as indicators of good dealer husbandry. The fish should not be desperately crowded – if they are it means that physical damage is more likely and parasites more easily transferred. Secondly, there should be some form of aeration and the fish should not be at the surface gasping for breath. Thirdly, there should be a water flow, preferably with filtration, if any of the water is recirculated. Failing to filter circulated

A common tapeworm of coarse fish: Ligula intestinalis. This tapeworm, shown in the upper fish, may equal the total weight of the fish

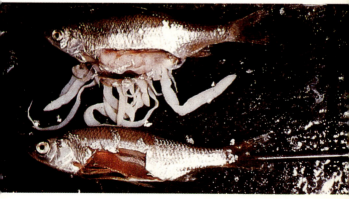

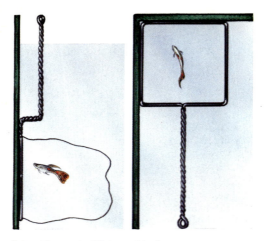

Careful netting out of fish avoids damage

water results in all fish batches being exposed to all the fish diseases present in the tanks in the system. Ideally all tanks should be independently provided with water and individually filtered. Finally there should be no ulcerated or badly-damaged fish, no dead or dying fish present in the set-up.

Quarantining new fish

To make absolutely sure that the fish you buy do not infect the rest of your fish with parasites or diseases you should always quarantine them first.

Quarantining allows the fish-keeper to observe new fish to ensure that they look healthy and behave normally. It also allows the fish to recover from the trauma of being transported without interference from other fish. Fish should be quarantined for three weeks. It is a very good idea to give two chemical treatments for external parasites at this stage, one near the beginning and one near the end of the quarantine period. You should not start to feed the fish until the second week of quarantine.

The quarantine tank should provide plenty of well-aerated water and should be in a quiet corner away from bright lights. It should not be subjected to sudden temperature changes.

Quarantining, even with chemical treatments, cannot guarantee fish as completely healthy. There are, for example, internal tapeworms and roundworms which have long life-cycles and which would not show up in three weeks. Knowing where and what sort of establishment the fish were bred at is an enormous help in trying to minimize these sorts of problems.

Occasionally, even after careful quarantining, new fish introduced into a tank or pond die within a few weeks. New, stressed fish may be attacked by infections to which your established stock have become resistant.

A healthy environment

Like other animals, fish suffer from many different diseases and some of them can kill. Fish are much more susceptible to diseases if they are in a bad condition. Poor water quality and unsuitable food are two of the commonest causes of poor condition in fish.

A fish living in a river, lake or the sea normally has several different parasitic animals living on or inside it. In natural conditions little harm is done to the fish by them. When fish are put into an overcrowded aquarium or pond, or one with a poor environment, parasites can

A typical small, balanced aquarium with built-in lighting

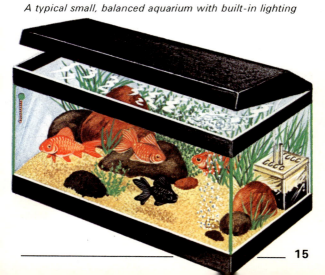

increase in numbers causing the fish to become 'diseased'. Apart from the density of fish making it easier for parasites to move from fish to fish, stress, often caused by careless handling or poor water quality, makes them prone to parasite infections.

To keep your fish healthy you must give them healthy surroundings. The most important ways of doing this are to give them enough room, keep them at the right temperature, keep their water well oxygenated and prevent their waste products (and decaying food) from building up.

Ponds and tanks

The first stage of keeping your fish healthy is to give them a sufficiently large home. This means buying a tank or digging a pond that is big enough and is the right shape. As a general rule fish up to 10 cm in length need at least 2 litres of water each, fish twice this size, 20 cm long, need at least 10 litres of water each and fish 30 cm long 50 litres ($3\frac{1}{2}$ pints for 4-inch, 2 gallons for 8-inch and 11 gallons for 12-inch fish). As you can see, big fish require considerably more water in proportion to their size than small fish. If you can afford it give each fish more than the minimum amount of space.

The proportions of the tank or pond are also important. You should aim to have the greatest possible water surface in relation to the volume of water. The greater the surface area of the pond the more easily oxygen can diffuse into the water. You should make sure that the

Larger fish require disproportionately more water

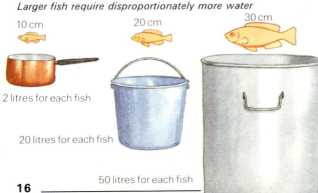

10 cm

20 cm

30 cm

2 litres for each fish

20 litres for each fish

50 litres for each fish

tank is not more than half as deep as it is long. A very deep tank has a small surface area in relation to its volume and will take up oxygen slowly. However, if you intend to aerate the tank with airstones deep tanks are an advantage as they allow the oxygen in the air bubbles more time to dissolve in the water as the bubbles rise to the surface.

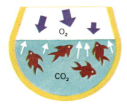

If you overcrowd the fish, oxygen in the atmosphere will not dissolve into the water quickly enough to meet their needs, and they will die. Overcrowding also slows their growth rate and may cause problems with pollution

Water
Sources
It is best to add a mixture of half rainwater and half tapwater to your new tank, if you can get clean rainwater.

Tapwater is not always a good source of water for a tank or pond. Chlorine added to tapwater to kill bacteria that are harmful to humans can unfortunately also kill fish. Usually most of the chlorine will have evaporated from the water by the time it reaches your tap (it will have done its job of killing bacteria by then) so it should be safe for fish. Even then it is best to let the water stand for at least 24 hours, so that you can be sure that all the chlorine has evaporated, before you put fish in it.

Water authorities also sometimes need to purge the water supply system with alkalis or insecticides. These are normally siphoned off but small concentrations may remain which are injurious to fish, so when tanks or ponds are refilled with water affected in this way, fish health problems may result.

However, if you need a lot of water, to fill a pond for example, you may have to use tapwater.

Clean rainwater is particularly good for many tropical

fish which require soft, slightly acid water. Water that is soft has a little calcium dissolved in it. Cold-water exotic fish, such as goldfish, can tolerate harder water with more calcium dissolved in it.

Pond or river water is not a good source of water. Parasites of fish will almost certainly be introduced if you use such water and although these may have little effect in the wild, in confined surroundings they may become much more abundant. Snails, insects and crustaceans that live in ponds and rivers can also carry fish parasites, so care should be taken not to introduce them with water or weeds by accident.

Water temperature

Different species and breeds of fish thrive at different water temperatures: some fish can live in seawater that is below 0°C (32°F); cold-water exotic fish, like koi and goldfish, can tolerate outdoor life in ponds; while all tropical fish need warm water all year round.

Allowing the temperature of a tropical fish aquarium to fall below 15°C (59°F) may kill the fish. You must make sure that you keep your fish at the temperature recommended.

All fish are cold-blooded, however, and on a cold day your goldfish or koi will be less active than on a warm day. In cold weather the metabolism of fish in outdoor ponds slows down. They use less oxygen, need less food and are generally less active.

Fish can be killed by temperatures outside their normal range

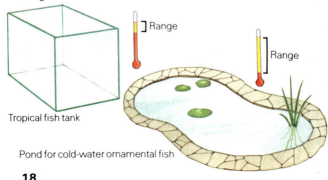

Tropical fish tank

Pond for cold-water ornamental fish

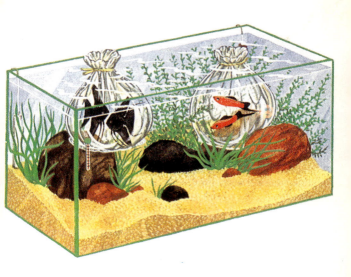

When you buy any fish, always float them in their unopened plastic bags for about 20 minutes: this equalizes the temperature between the bag and aquarium and avoids distressing the fish when released

Although the surface of outdoor ponds may freeze over in winter, only in exceptionally harsh winters will the water at the bottom of the pond fall below 4°C (40°F). This temperature can also be reached in unheated sheds and on single-glazed window sills. Normally 4°C is therefore regarded as the absolute minimum. In the height of summer ponds may reach 26–28°C (78–83°F), and indoor aquariums exposed to the sun even more – perhaps 30°C (86°F). So over the year a cold-blooded fish will change its body temperature from 4°C to 28°C. The reactions of a fish at 4°C are totally different from those of one at 28°C.

Temperature fluctuations There are important differences between fish kept at a constant temperature and those kept at seasonal or semi-seasonal temperatures; fish of the carp family need increased temperature to mature. If the temperatures do not vary they may develop eggs or sperm to an intermediate stage, but

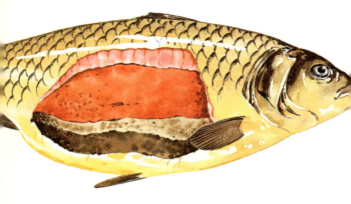

Large numbers of eggs are produced by members of the carp family when environmental conditions are suitable

will not complete their sexual development. Carp, for example, need minimum temperatures of 21°C for several days before they will spawn and will only spawn then if the previous temperatures have been high enough. The maturity of other families of fish may depend on temperature or day length.

If fish like carp, goldfish, orfe or tench develop to an intermediate stage, but do not spawn, they may have considerable difficulties in coping with their development, particularly the females. This can cause death of the fish – it is a common problem in goldfish and koi.

Of course you will not be able to keep your fish at a temperature that is always the same, especially if they are in an outdoor pond. Then you must remember that fish will tolerate slow changes of temperature much more easily than fast ones. One of the main reasons why many goldfish and other cold-water exotic fish are sold in such poor condition in early spring and summer is that they have been kept in small display tanks outdoors and have experienced temperature changes of 10°C (18°F) or more in a day. Such changes put the fish under stress, which lowers their natural resistance to all kinds of parasites and diseases. So one of the most important aspects of being a good fish-keeper is to keep stressful changes in their environment to a minimum.

Fish, being cold blooded, adopt their surrounding temperature and when temperatures drop, their rate of body activity, including defence against infection, decreases. In really cold conditions it may almost cease. However, slow swimming and respiration still result in minor cuts which bacteria viruses and fungi invade. In the intestine damage may be due to rough food, in the gills to sharp suspended solids, and on the body surface to the fish bumping into sharp objects. When warm weather arrives activity starts to increase. The bacteria, and other small organisms multiply quite rapidly. The fish, however, being relatively large, takes quite some time to regain their defence mechanisms, which can lead to severe infection.

This is much more likely to happen if the rise in temperature is rapid: a slow increase in temperature allows the fish's reactions to improve at a rate which can control the bacterial increase.

Small tanks and ponds have relatively small thermal capacities and so can heat up and cool down rapidly compared with larger bodies of water. If this happens

'Pinecone' effect seen in dropsy

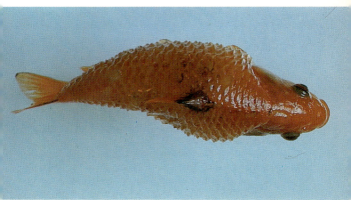

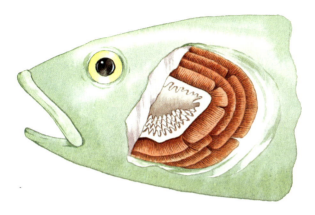

*Inside the gill cover (*operculum*) there are four double gills on each side*

repeatedly over a short period, like a day and night, the fish will start to show symptoms of temperature stress and will slowly lose condition, eventually dying. With small tanks insulation or thermostatically-controlled water heaters (or both) can eliminate these sorts of difficulties.

Aim for changes in water temperature of no more than 2°C a day and your fish will be less likely to suffer from thermal stress. Another good reason for having as large a tank or pond as you can afford is that the greater the volume of water you have the more slowly its temperature will change.

Water composition

Your fish require a constant supply of oxygen. They get this from the water which they pump over their gills. Watch your fish breathing. Like us they breathe instinctively, taking gulps of water just as we take gulps of air. Every time the gill cover opens and closes the fish has taken a breath.

There is far less oxygen in water than in air (about 1/10,000th as much) and it is quite common for fish to die of lack of oxygen, especially in small tanks and ponds where there is a very small reserve of oxygen.

The greater the volume of water you have for each fish the less chance there is that your fish will run out of oxygen.

Another problem with the supply of oxygen is that the warmer the water becomes the less oxygen it contains. At 20°C (68°F) there is about half the amount of oxygen than there is at 10°C (50°F). To make things worse fish (and any other plant or animal in the water) use more oxygen as they warm up. So you will see that, at least out of doors, summer can be a very difficult time of the year for the fish – there is less oxygen in the water and they are using it more rapidly.

Unless you have an oxygen meter it is very difficult to know how much oxygen there is in the water. One pointer is to watch your fish in warm weather: if they are spending a lot of time near the surface gasping they may be short of oxygen. Other symptoms of lack of oxygen are crowding under a fountain or at a water inlet and general sluggishness.

The same symptoms occur if, for some reason, a fish's gills or blood system are not working properly. So if you are sure that there is copious oxygen available and the fish are gasping turn your attention to gill problems or blood problems.

Fish, water and the other organisms in the water need to be in harmony

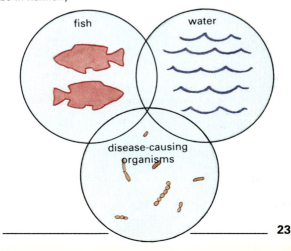

fish

water

disease-causing organisms

THE HEALTHY AQUARIUM

Aeration Unless you have very few fish in a large tank you should always aerate the water. Aerating the water not only oxygenates it but also removes carbon dioxide and other gases produced by the fish as waste products of their metabolism.

There are many different kinds of aerator available but ensure that you choose one that is powerful enough to suit your size of tank. Break up the air bubbles as they enter the water with an airstone. The small bubbles created by the airstone aerate the water more efficiently than large bubbles. As the fish use up the oxygen in the water it is replaced by oxygen in the air bubbles rising up through the water. If you keep fish in a pond out of doors fit a small fountain as this will also help to oxygenate the water. Planting oxygenating plants also helps.

External filter   Box filter

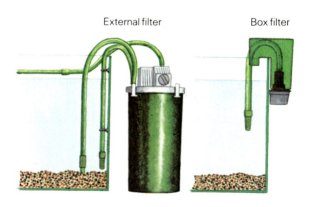

Power filters enable the number of fish kept in an aquarium to be increased. They are of several different types

Ammonia
Fish are not only affected by the amount of oxygen in the water. Other chemicals dissolved in water can also affect the health of your fish. One of the most important of these is ammonia, which is produced by the kidneys of fish as a waste product.

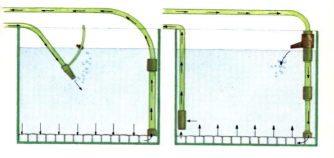

Filters, such as the under-gravel filter shown above, provide a large surface area on which beneficial bacteria live

It is very toxic and must be excreted into the water. In lakes, rivers and the sea there is usually so much water to dilute the ammonia produced by fish that it never reaches a concentration that is dangerous, unless the water is polluted. In a small tank or pond, however, there is far less water available to dilute the ammonia and it may be sufficiently concentrated to be harmful to the fish.

Ammonia has several effects, including causing permanent damage to the gills. The gills of fish that have been exposed to high levels of ammonia have a much reduced surface area so that breathing is much less efficient.

Because of this many tanks and ponds have filters which break down ammonia.

Filtration   Bacteria which convert ammonia into less toxic matter will do this job for you. The filter may be either inside or outside the tank. The most important feature of the filter is that it should contain a material with a very large surface area, such as synthetic cotton-wool or angular gravel. These materials have space for the many millions of bacteria that break down the ammonia and other waste products. You must re-member that these bacteria also use up oxygen so that water coming out of a filter needs aeration before it is returned to the tank or pond.

In tanks and ponds, particularly marine tanks and biologically filtered ponds, salts derived from ammonia can cause problems to fish. Different fish species tolerate different levels, but inevitably in closed recirculation systems these may be exceeded. Symptoms are listlessness, gasping, hanging near the surface, gill congestion and death. Testing kits are available to check these levels. If a biological filter is used in a recirculated aquarium or pond there will be a brief rise in the nitrite level for the first few days or weeks after installation. This is quite normal: the process should adjust itself after the first few days.

Biological filters should be treated as living creatures. If they are kept short of food (i.e. fish wastes) they will grow more slowly, if they are heavily loaded they will develop very quickly. Both states are quite acceptable, but rapid changes from little fish waste to a great deal of fish waste and vice versa will create problems for the filter and it will not work well. It should also be remembered that filters work more slowly in cold weather. When renewing the gravel or sand in a biological filter many fish-keepers transfer a small quantity of old material to the new filter. This is to 'seed' the new filter with the right groups of bacteria and speed up its development.

Filters encourage the breakdown of ammonia. They also keep the water clear of suspended particles. Bacteria are almost certain to be growing on these suspended particles and if there is a great deal of suspended material in the water the bacteria may use up a large amount of the oxygen in the tank or pond. These bacteria are also likely to be a source of infection for the fish.

Correct feeding
Quantities

The commonest mistake in feeding fish is to give them too much food. Adult fish require only little more than a 100th of their body weight of dry food every day. For a 10 cm (4-inch) long fish, weighing about 10 grams, you need to feed only 0.1 gram every day. A fish of 20 cm (8 inches), weighing about 100 grams (4 oz), would need about a gram of food every day.

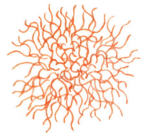

a mass of red *Tubifex* worms

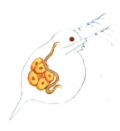

vigorously swimming
water fleas (Daphnia)

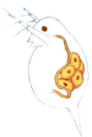

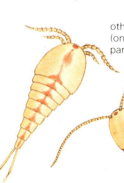

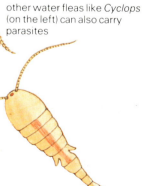

other water fleas like *Cyclops*
(on the left) can also carry
parasites

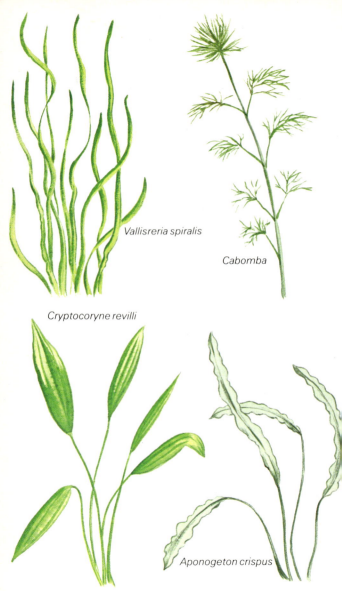

Vallisreria spiralis

Cabomba

Cryptocoryne revilli

Aponogeton crispus

All these plants are suitable for a well-lit, healthy aquarium

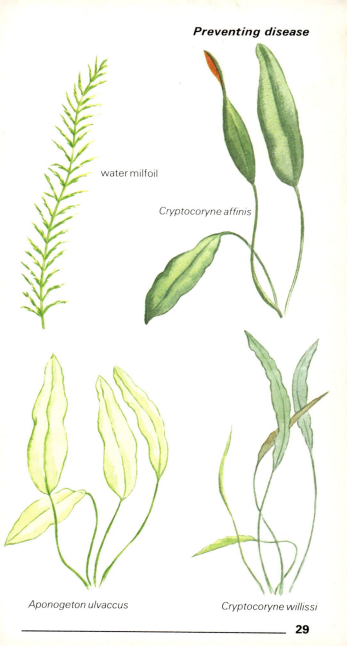

water milfoil

Cryptocoryne affinis

Aponogeton ulvaccus

Cryptocoryne willissi

When fish eat dried foods they have to drink water to moisten them before digestion. Although there is some variation between different dried foods, as a general rule there is a tenfold increase in the weight of dried food on hydration.

It is important not to overfeed your fish. If given the opportunity, fish will eat much more food than they need. Once fish have reached their maximum size overfeeding often results in them accumulating large amounts of fat around their internal organs. It is quite normal for fish to store excess food as fat. In natural conditions this would be consumed during the winter and early spring when the fish were not feeding. In tropical fish it would be consumed in the non-productive seasons when food was scarce. Some fish store fat in the liver, others as a separate fat body. In cultured or pet fish where there is no distinct winter, the fat accumulation is never utilized and can lead to problems of overweight. Accumulated fat can prevent fish from spawning and may be deposited around the heart blocking its blood supply.

Types of food

Fish eat a great variety of different foods in the wild. Some feed on plants, some on aquatic invertebrates, some on other fish. However, most common aquarium fish can be fed on flaked foods.

It is worth remembering that fish are naturally adapted to feed on different kinds of foods. Fish of the carp family (the cyprinids), for example, often feed on detritus and decaying plant material. They have digestive systems designed to process large amounts of poor quality food. Presented with too much protein-rich food they can become obese.

Live foods

If you want to give fish live food make sure you give plants to fish that are naturally herbivorous and animals to fish that are naturally carnivorous.

Live foods are good for fish but may endanger their health if the food has come from the wild. Several common live foods, such as *Daphnia*, *Cyclops* and *Tubifex*, can carry the immature stages of some fish

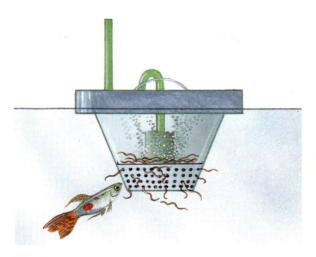

The advantages of feeding live food must be balanced with the disadvantages

parasites. When the fish eats an infected animal it in turn becomes infected. If a lot of food animals carry parasites the fish may become heavily infected as it eats more live food.

It is quite easy to culture living food for fish. Most of the life cycles of the common food organisms are fairly simple and can be maintained in simple aquariums or pots. A rainwater butt is very useful for culturing *Daphnia, Cyclops* or mosquito larvae which can be cropped for up to eight months of the year. During the winter months, heated systems are required to produce them. For algal eaters the process is even easier for most water left in a greenhouse or indoors exposed to the air and light will produce an algal bloom. Seeding and fertilizer will increase the yield enormously. Food organisms reared in this way do not harbour parasites dangerous to the fish.

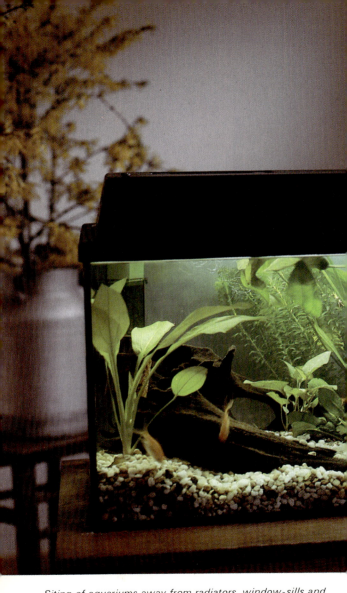

Siting of aquariums away from radiators, window-sills and draughts, is important

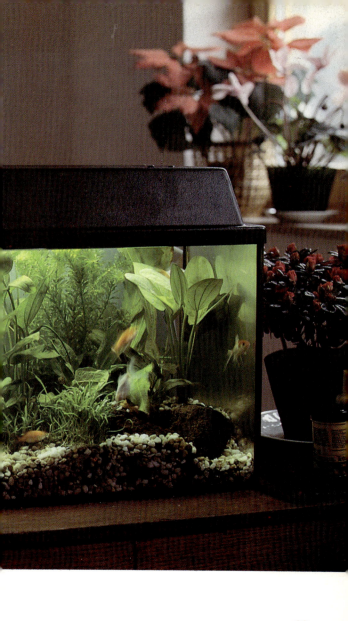

Fish
diseases

Causes

Some fish diseases are caused by poor water quality, some by inadequate feeding, others by bacteria, viruses, fungi and parasites and yet others by physical damage or genetic inheritance. Frequently in fish it is a combination of all these factors.

Rough handling will encourage diseases by damaging the fish's skin, as well as removing the layer of mucus that is the fish's first protection against bacteria, viruses and parasites. Damaged skin often leads to secondary infections caused by bacteria.

A fish's skin is a living tissue, unlike human skin which has an accumulation of dead cells overlying the living cells. It has several important functions in fish such as breathing, getting rid of soluble waste, streamlining and camouflage. Any problem that affects the skin affects all these functions and therefore has consequences in other parts and functions of the fish.

Typical examples of severe fin erosion and ulceration

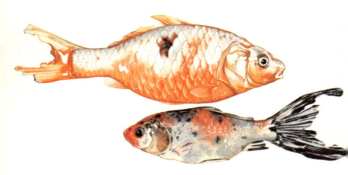

Parasites

Many of the common diseases of ornamental fish are caused by a small number of common parasitic animals that live on the outside of the fish. Most of the parasites

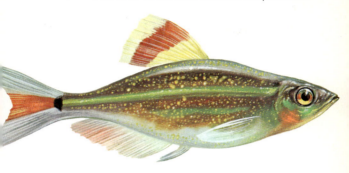

White Cloud Mountain Minnow suffering from Velvet Disease: body covered with light-brown dust-like parasites

How to prevent infection spreading in a tank

possible carriers of infection

do not transfer from infected to healthy tanks

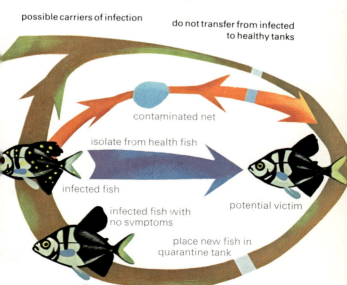

contaminated net

isolate from health fish

infected fish

potential victim

infected fish with no symptoms

place new fish in quarantine tank

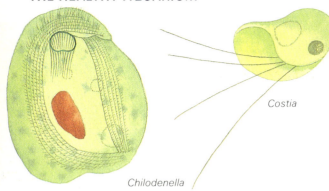

Costia

Chilodenella

Two common external parasites, Chilodonella *and* Costia

and other organisms that cause diseases in fish are very small and can only be seen under the microscope.

Parasites which do not need other animals to complete their life-cycle but which spread directly from fish to fish are the most dangerous to ornamental fish.

Trichodina; *another very common skin parasite*

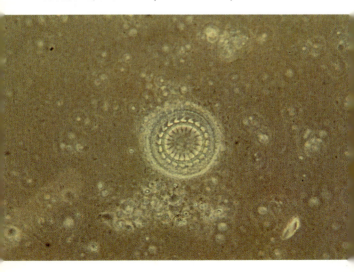

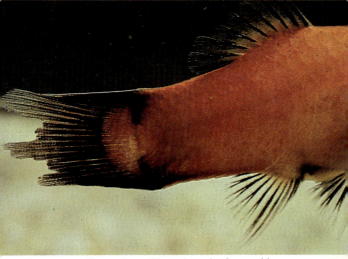

Even severe fin-erosion will repair under favourable conditions

Symptoms

Damaged fins Several common parasites damage the fins of fish. When many are present on the fish the fins may become quite ragged and often have many small red blotches on them. These are areas where the parasites have broken the blood vessels in the fin, causing it to bleed very slightly. Three single-celled parasites that commonly cause these symptoms are *Costia*, *Chilodonella* and *Trichodina*.

White spots The commonest parasite affecting ornamental fish has the almost impossibly long scientific name of *Ichthyophthirius multifiliis*. Not surprisingly most people call it White Spot after the symptoms of a heavy infection. White Spot probably causes the death of more ornamental fish than any other parasite or disease. Warm-water, cold-water, fresh-water and brackish water fish are all affected. It can spread directly between fish and can be transferred on nets, stones, water plants or by drops of water. It lives on the skin or gills of the fish where it grows up to 2 mm in diameter. It then falls off the fish and releases hundreds of larvae which go in search of other fish. Once they have found one they burrow under the skin where they live for a time before assuming the typical 'White Spot' appearance.

The whole process (the parasite's life-cycle) may take as much as two months at 7°C (44.6°F) or as little as five to six days at 25°C (77°F). Low levels of White Spot may exist in a tank for years, only developing into an epidemic after some traumatic event such as the introduction of new fish or a rapid change in water temperature or water chemistry.

White Spot was formerly regarded as a fish parasite which either produced the distinctive symptoms or lived as a larval phase for up to 48 hours away from the fish. Therefore theoretically it should have been possible, by removing fish from the water, to create a White Spot-free pond. If the fish were treated at the same time, the problem should have been solved. In fact White Spot is one of the most difficult parasites to get rid of. It appears that there are different strains that take different amounts of time to complete their life

Whitespot: the commonest fish-killing disease of all

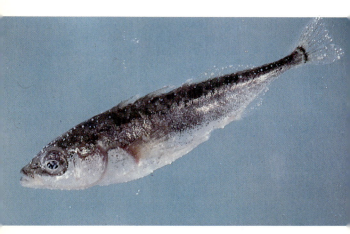

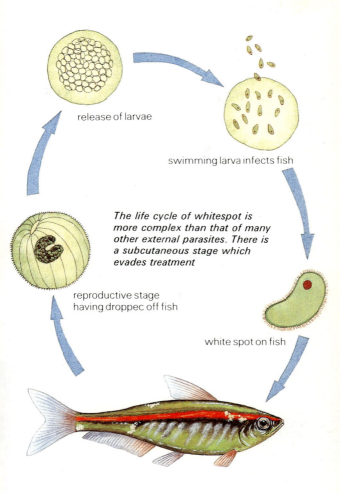

release of larvae

swimming larva infects fish

The life cycle of whitespot is more complex than that of many other external parasites. There is a subcutaneous stage which evades treatment

reproductive stage having dropped off fish

white spot on fish

cycle and that the amount of time is also dependent on host-species as well as temperature. So what was thought of originally as a simple problem has proved much more complex to solve.

The loss of scales associated with this may lead to secondary infections by bacteria and fungi.

Listlessness and emaciation   Any parasite present in a heavy infection is likely to make fish thin and listless. However, two blood-sucking parasites are especially likely to do this. Both are distant relatives of crabs and belong to the group of animals called crustaceans. The two parasites are the fish louse and the gill louse. The fish louse lives on many different species of fish but cold-water exotics are probably the most susceptible. It is saucer-shaped, can be as much as 12mm ($\frac{1}{2}$ inch) long and is most abundant in September and October. It feeds on skin cells and blood and, if several are present on one fish, it can cause anaemia. It can swim from fish to fish but usually the weakest fish in a tank is preferred.

There are 200 species of fish louse worldwide which affect a wide range of fish in South America, Asia, Europe and Australasia. Imported fish may carry them with them. Most species are capable of infecting a wide range of fish hosts, so whole communities of fish can be affected.

An unrelated group of parasites which has similar effects are leeches. They are blood suckers which make

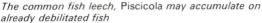

The common fish leech, Piscicola *may accumulate on already debilitated fish*

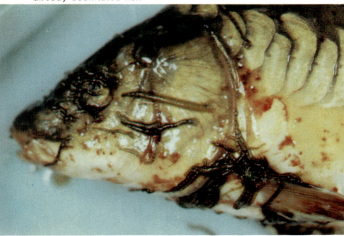

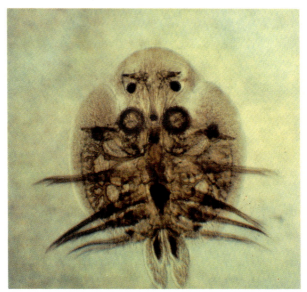

Attachment by Argulus *is by the two circular suckers seen above*

holes and cause bleeding in fish, resulting in anaemia. Anaemia in fish is indicated by slow gasping, and very pale gills. Although rarely directly fatal, it weakens the fish, making it prey to secondary bacterial and fungal problems.

Rubbing on tank sides Many parasites irritate the skin of the fish. Naturally the fish try to get rid of the irritation and rubbing themselves on the sides of the tank is one way in which they try to do this.

Sliminess The irritation also causes the fish to produce extra mucus making the fish appear more slimy than normal. 'Grey-slime', 'blue-slime' and 'white-slime' are all names used to describe this condition. Excessive slime or mucus is a reaction to infection or irritation by the fish. Mucus provides a protective layer and is mildly antibiotic. However, in

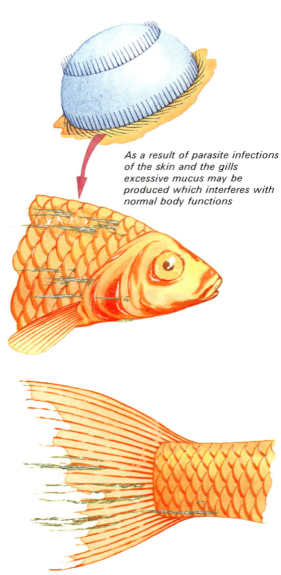

As a result of parasite infections of the skin and the gills excessive mucus may be produced which interferes with normal body functions

large quantities it can be harmful to the fish's health in some ways. For example, thicker mucus slows down the functioning of the skin and the gills particularly. In really exceptional cases excessive mucus may seriously impair the fish's breathing. Rubbing and slime are a sign of a heavy infection with parasites like *Costia*, *Chilodonella*, *Trichodina* or White Spot.

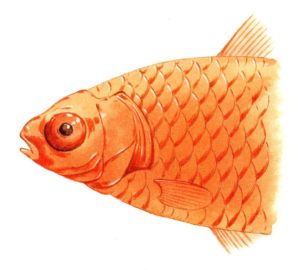

Many of the symptoms of sick fish in freshwater reflect kidney failure and retention of water

Pop-eyes, bloating, raised scales *Costia, Trichodina* and *Chilodonella* are all single-celled animals that live on the skin and gills of fish. They affect a wide range of fresh-water fish and there are different species that grow at different temperatures. They feed on the fish's skin and mucus and may remove the surface layers completely. Without a sound barrier of skin, the kidney has to work, possibly to the point of failing, to keep an ideal balance of body water and dissolved salts.

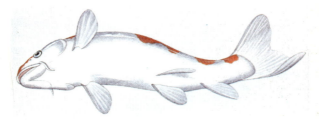

Fish with skin parasites often swim erratically, 'flashing' with their undersides

Flashing Many fish are camouflaged by being darkly-coloured on the back and lighter on the belly. Looking down on fish from above, the dark colour is difficult to see against the dark background of the water. From below, the white belly of the fish is difficult to see against the light from the sky.

The irritation caused by skin parasites often makes fish swim erratically, turning their light undersides upwards making them very conspicuous. This 'flashing' may help the parasites to find the next host in their life-cycle by making the fish more obvious to their predators like herons and cormorants. White Spot and all the protozoan parasites can cause fish to 'flash'.

When fish are short of oxygen they swim sluggishly at the surface gasping for air

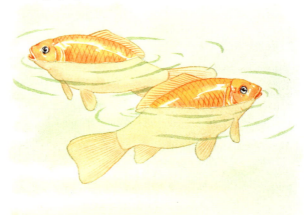

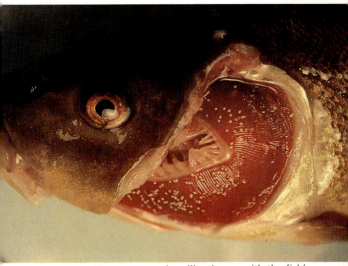

Ergasilus *the gill maggot on the gills, shown with the fish's gill cover removed*

Gasping Several common skin parasites can also live on the gills of fish. Gill flukes (like *Dactylogyrus*) and White Spot are both able to live on the gills where they can do great damage. The gill louse is one of the most dangerous parasites for semi-tropical and cold-water fish and feeds on blood in the gills. It is free-living through most of its life-cycle and is unlikely to survive this free-living stage in a pond or tank. However, once infected, fish are at risk.

There are several species of *Ergasilus* and related forms that occur worldwide. Therefore it is possible to import fish which already have an infection. It is difficult to treat and fish with relatively high numbers suffer from anaemia and gill-damage.

All these parasites irritate the gill tissue causing the fish to make much more mucus than it would do normally. The extra mucus prevents oxygen from diffusing from the water into the blood vessels of the gills and to get more oxygen the fish comes nearer to the surface and may even try to 'breathe' air. The

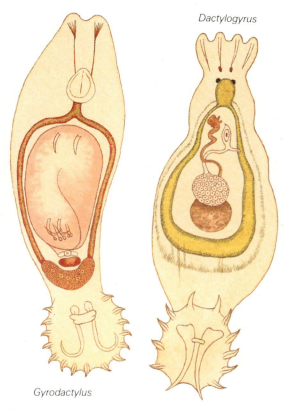

Dactylogyrus

Gyrodactylus

The two commonest flukes, Dactylogyrus *with eyespots and* Gyrodactylus *with young larva developing inside*

parasites also destroy gill tissue directly; *Dactylogyrus*, for example, has anchor-shaped hooks at the hind end which it digs into the gill filaments. *Dactylogyrus* can spread from fish to fish as it has a swimming larval stage.

It is known as a direct life cycle parasite, there being no other hosts involved in the life cycle – only the fish. This means that infection levels in community tanks can build up relatively easily and quickly.

Tattered fins   *Gyrodactylus* is often a cause of fin erosion. It lives a similar existence to *Dactylogyrus* but its main centre of infection is the fin, particularly the tail fin and anal fin. Its presence in large numbers is characterized by an erosion of the fin margins, a general 'tattiness' and blood-flecks appearing throughout the fin rays.

Fungi, bacteria and viruses

There are some bacteria that are cold-water forms, some that exist at intermediate temperatures and those that only cause problems in warm-water fish. Fish tuberculosis is caused by a bacterium that is a warm-water form. It is not uncommonly found in imports of tropical fish. There are also bacteria of marine fish that create enormous problems.

There are several conditions of fish that produce white spots. Most can be treated in a similar way. This Chanda ranga *has velvet*

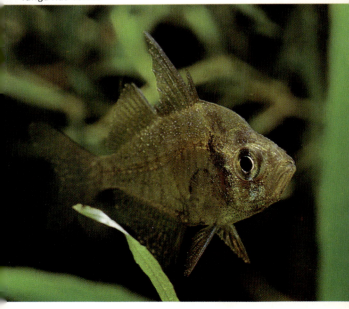

Symptoms

Ulcers Ulcers which expose the flesh of the fish are a particularly unpleasant sight. They can form almost anywhere on the body and are usually the result of a bacterial infection. Infections by bacteria often follow damage to the skin either by rough handling or following an attack by skin parasites.

Ulcers may result from fish lice, leeches or from physical damage which makes the fish vulnerable to bacteria infection.

A bacterial ulcer has a central area where the bacteria have killed the fish tissue and where the tissue will appear white or may have disappeared leaving a pronounced hole. Around this central area will be a ring of red, slightly swollen, inflamed tissue where the fish is

A typical bacterial ulcer

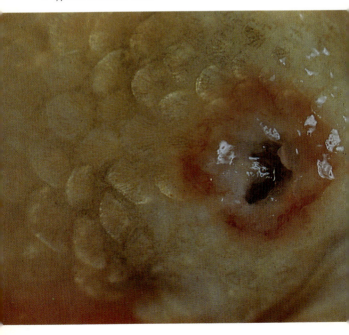

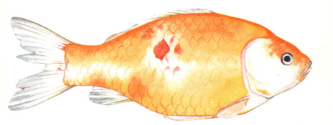

Ulcers are often caused by secondary bacterial infections after an attack by skin parasites

fighting the infection. Further out still the tissue is normal and shows no signs of any disease problem. Once a bacterial ulcer has started it has three possible outcomes: it may heal itself, worsen, in which case the fish will eventually die, or it may persist unchanged. In this last case the balance can often be tipped in favour of the fish by improving its environment.

Some bacteria start the disease from inside the fish. In these cases ulcers or broken blood vessels may suddenly appear on different parts of the body in a relatively short time. Fish in this condition should be separated from the rest of your fish in a tank on their own. If fish develop these symptoms you may need to call in a professional fish pathologist to make an examination.

Bloatedness This is most frequently caused by *Aeromonas hydrophila*, which affects the kidney, causing fluid retention or dropsy. It normally affects fish when water temperatures are above 15°C (59°F).

Bleeding Bacterial ulcers of marine fish at relatively high temperatures (above 20°C, 68°F), particularly in low strength sea water are frequently caused by the bacterium *Vibrio anguillarum*. The condition it causes, Vibriosis, is often called Redpest, because of the large areas of haemorrhage that can be seen on the surface of infected fish.

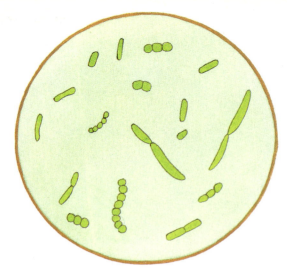

Bacteria of several different types can be seen on the skin of even healthy fish with the aid of a powerful microscope

Carp with abdominal dropsy

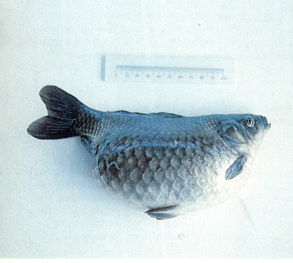

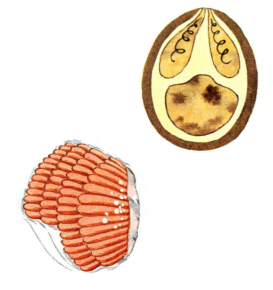

White cysts on gills. The gill cover has been removed
Right: *the cysts' spore greatly enlarged*

Infected gills Another very common disease caused by bacteria affects the gills of the fish. Called myxobacterial gill disease, it usually affects fish if the water is badly filtered and contains a lot of suspended particles and decaying matter. Fish gasp for oxygen at the surface of the water with this disease and trails of thick brown mucus can be seen hanging from the gills and sometimes from the pectoral fins.

White 'cotton-wool' on the skin or gills The appearance of a greyish-white 'cotton-wool' on the skin or gills of the fish shows that it is suffering from an infection of the fungus *Saprolegnia*. *Saprolegnia* grows on the skin and gills when the water is not properly filtered or the skin of the fish has been damaged. It can grow on dead tissue, including dead food, so it is important to keep the tank free from this sort of debris.

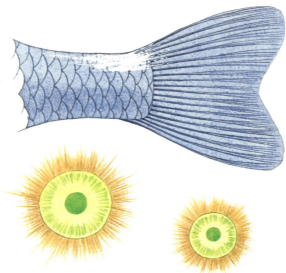

The cotton-wool fungus and its spore Saprolegnia *grows on most organic matter, such as live fish or dead eggs*

White lumps on the skin Solid white lumps, several millimetres across, often appear on the skin of fish of the carp family. These growths are called carp pox, caused by a virus, and are commonest when the water is cold. They are usually harmless, cannot be treated, but disappear as the water warms up.

There is some debate about whether non-carp family fish in cold conditions can contract this virus. Some races of koi from hot climates are much more susceptible to outbreaks of carp pox than those from colder climates. The fish louse can transmit this infection from fish to fish and it is also possible for people to transmit it with nets or on hands. The impressions of fingers of carp-pox on the backs of large carp have been recorded because of fish farmers handling infected, then non-infected fish under cold conditions.

Like many fish and other animal viruses carp pox, once with a fish, is with it for life. Although the symptoms may disappear as the water is warmed up, the virus as a latent infection will still be present.

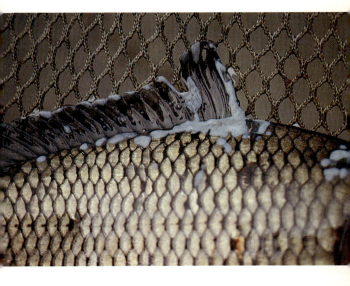

This is the most typical appearance of carp pox with hard white translucent patches of various sizes. Sometimes these patches are softer and slightly red

Other causes of fish ailments
Gas pressure

Green plants produce oxygen during the day, but consume it during the night. Too many plants in a tank or pond can lead to a sharp decline in oxygen concentration at night. This may cause the gas to rush out of the tissues so rapidly that it forms bubbles causing bleeding, disorientation, and, in severe cases, death. A similar effect can be produced by an intermittent air leak in a pump or a powered filter. Bubbles of gas trapped in the fins, in the eyes and in the gills are the tell-tale symptoms of this and the cure is to remove the cause of the variation of gas pressure. In the case of plant-related gas problems reducing the number of plants or constant light levels would suffice; with intermittent air leaks repairing or replacing the system is called for.

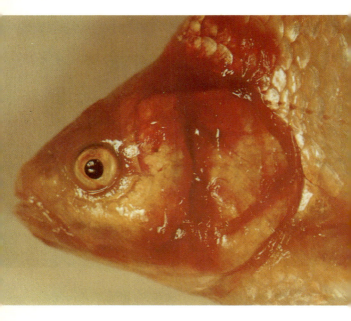

Gas bubble disease results in the bursting of many small blood vessels producing an angry-looking bleeding area

Poisoning

Aquarists and pond-keepers are great innovators and use many novel devices composed of many different materials. Some of these materials (non-aquariumastic, non-standard butyl liners. pumps with brass or copper connectors) may under certain circumstances produce disastrous results. So if you are planning to use a novel material, investigate its toxicity to fish by enquiring from your supplier or the manufacturers.

Sprays used on houseplants and in the garden represent another well known source of poison to fish, but less well known and equally dangerous are some of the paints and polishes used domestically or in do-it-yourself projects. Over such chemicals the advice has to be – if in doubt keep it away from your fish system.

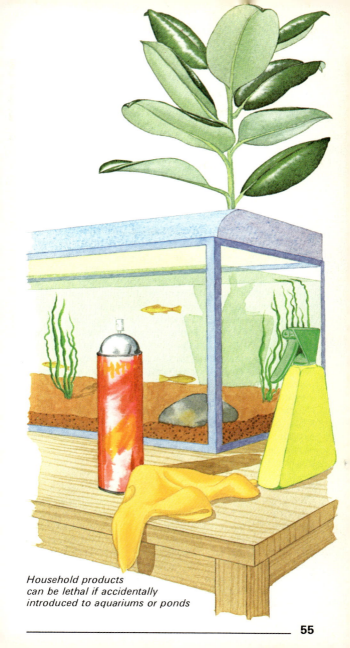

*Household products
can be lethal if accidentally
introduced to aquariums or ponds*

Simple treatments for diseased fish

Substances

To treat diseased fish you will need a small range of chemicals. You must always be careful with these chemicals because they can be dangerous to people and animals. Do not leave any of your fish 'medicines' near the fish tank; keep them in a secure cupboard.

There are five chemical compounds that you may need to treat your fish: formalin, malachite green, salt, acriflavine and chloramine T. There are, of course, a variety of proprietary brands that incorporate these chemicals. Although more expensive, many of these are the result of extensive studies that have aimed to maximize effectiveness and minimize risk. With such a wide choice of chemicals, you can afford to be very particular about which brand you choose. It is advisable to select that which provides you with the maximum amount of information concerning the contents or at least the active ingredients and which explains most fully the conditions in which the material works best, its limitations and the range of safety for treating fish for the parasites or problems described.

Formalin should be used to treat White Spot, *Costia*, *Chilodonella*, *Trichodina*. When treating White Spot you should add a few drops of malachite green to the formalin. Formalin (as the chemical compound 40 per cent formaldehyde) is sold by agricultural suppliers and chemists for use as a sterilizing agent. It is strongly acidic so great care must be taken when using it, either by buffering it with a teaspoon of sodium bicarbonate (baking powder) to reduce the acidity or by giving a salt bath afterwards. As formalin removes the oxygen from water, aeration should always be given during treatment. If white spot is suspected a second treatment must be given four to five days later.

Salt is normally sold with additives that allow it to run freely. A common running agent is sodium hexacyanate which can be toxic to fish, especially when used as a long term bath. Salt sold in bulk in garden centres for de-icing your garden paths contains other chemicals so it is important to obtain the pure product. If a large quantity is required it is a good idea to buy from a chemical supplier. Sea-salt (from health shops) is also a good source.

Acriflavine The third chemical you may need is acriflavine which should be applied as a general antiseptic to wounds and sores. Acriflavine can be bought from any large chemical manufacturer in powder form (which is orange-red). It is a chemical that makes fish hypersensitive to sunlight and should always be used in subdued light. It has been used to kill myxobacteria and protozoans and to assist wound repair. Like formalin, acriflavine can be very acid so some type of buffer should be incorporated into the treatment.

Chloramine T If you suspect that your fish have a bacterial infection of the gills they should be treated with chloramine T. This is obtainable in a liquid form from many chemists and is normally used as a bath.

Antibiotics You may also want to give the fish an antibiotic in its food if a bacterial infection has been diagnosed by a vet. You should not use antibiotics unless absolutely necessary. Many people carelessly (and illegally) use human antibiotics for fish. Although this may help their fish it may also encourage strains of bacteria that are resistant to these antibiotics, making them less useful for human medicine.

All chemicals used for treatment should be kept in sealed containers and at a constant (preferably low) temperature. Formalin, acriflavine, malachite green and chloramine T will deteriorate within 12 months if they are not kept in these conditions.

Techniques

There are three ways in which you can treat a sick fish. You can give it a *dip* by placing it in a strong solution of the treatment chemical for a very short time. You can given it a *bath* with a weaker solution for a longer time. Finally you can give it a *topical treatment*, applying a very concentrated medication to a wound or sore.

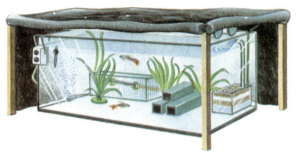

During convalescence fish should be kept in a quiet dimly-lit area

If you intend to treat several fish always try the treatment on one fish first. It is easy to make mistakes in making up the solutions and you may kill the fish you are trying to treat.

After treating fish for parasites you should put them into a recovery tank containing a mild solution of salt. You should add 5 grams of salt to every litre and continue to aerate the water vigorously. The fish should be kept in the recovery tank for 24 hours and should not be fed during that time.

Useful addresses

Association of Aquarists
Secretary
Mrs A. Ottley
71 St Michael's Road
Aldershot
Hampshire GU12 4JJ
(An association of over 50 aquarist societies in the
United Kingdom)

Confederation of Aquarists
Mr and Mrs W. Bennett
15 Coulter Avenue
Wishaw
Lanarkshire ML2 8SZ
Scotland
(An association of different specialist aquatic
societies in the United Kingdom)

Aquarist and Pondkeeper magazine (monthly)
The Butts
Half Acre
Brentford
Middlesex TW8 8BN

Practical Fishkeeper magazine (monthly)
Pursuit Publications Limited
Bretton Court
Bretton
Peterborough PE3 8DZ

Index

Photographic acknowledgments

Bruce Coleman – Hans Reinhard front cover, 32-33; Laurence E. Perkins 9; Hamlet Partnership 10, 13, 21, 36, 38, 40, 41, 45, 48, 50, 53, 54; Ian Sellick 37; Bill Tomey 47

Illustrations by Linden Artists Ltd (David Webb, Steve Lings and Colin Newman)